AF891633

A NURSES STORY

From Student Nurse to CEO
A journey in Aged Care

Susan Wray

ISBN: 978-1-7647247-1-5

NATIONAL LIBRARY OF AUSTRALIA

A catalogue record for this book is available from the National Library of Australia

© Copyright 2026 - All rights reserved.

It is not legal to reproduce, duplicate, or transmit any part of this document in either electronic means or printed format. Recording this publication is strictly prohibited.

mangwray.com

I dedicate this book to

My parents
who supported and encouraged me to become a Nurse, installing true values of respect, dignity and hard work.

Claire Schmierer
who inspired and mentored me to become the leader I am today

My family
who have come along for the ride, with support, love and many laughs at my expense.

This is for you all.

Table of Contents

Forward

Not all stories from the frontline of healthcare are told in hushed tones or clinical language. Some are raw, some are confronting, and some, unexpectedly, are darkly funny.

This book is a personal account of my journey, from student, to nurse, to CEO. It is a story shaped not only by care and compassion, but by resilience, humour, and the ability to endure a system that was often as challenging as the work itself. To protect privacy, many names have been changed, particularly those of residents, patients, and institutions. In some cases, I have referred only to broader geographical areas.

Along the way, there are moments I recount that may, at first glance, seem irreverent or even disrespectful. That is not my intention. These are the moments that, behind closed doors, made me laugh, lifted my spirit, and carried me through what was often a difficult and emotionally demanding profession, one made unnecessarily harder by layers of government bureaucracy and red tape.

I would like to acknowledge one person in particular who has shaped my journey: Claire Schmierer. A mentor and friend for more than 25 years, she was not only one of my original nursing lecturers but later became a close friend and profound influence on my leadership during my time in aged care. Her guidance left a lasting mark on who I am, both professionally and personally.

To my husband and children, thank you. You have listened patiently to my stories and endured countless dinner table conversations about bowel movements; a topic nurses seem endlessly fascinated by. Your support and humour have meant everything.

These pages reflect my personal memories, experiences, and opinions. At times, they will reveal instances of poor practice and lapses in ethics within the healthcare field. Thankfully, much has changed, and standards of care, knowledge, and professionalism have improved significantly over time.

If you recognise yourself in these stories, please understand that they are drawn from my own observations and recollections, shaped by the perspective and context of the time.

All photographs included in this book have been used with consent.

Susan Wray

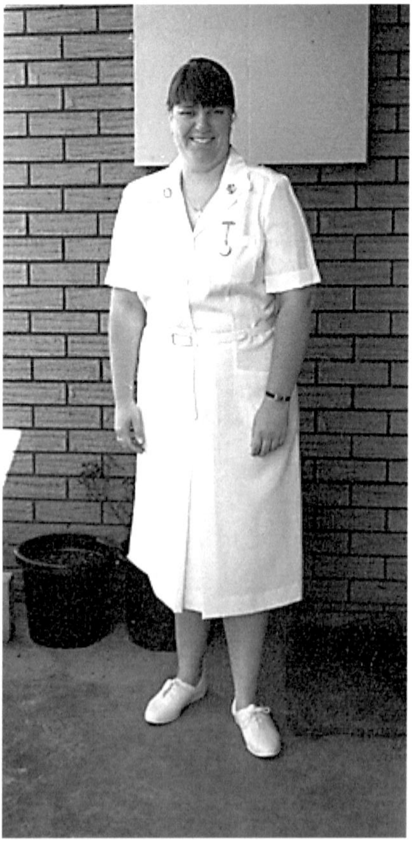

Chapter 1
Where It Began

Nursing was never my childhood dream. It wasn't something I declared at five years old or held onto through adolescence. Instead, it found me quietly and unexpectedly during my teenage years, when I volunteered as a first aider for local football teams. At the time, it felt incidental, just something I did. Looking back, it was the beginning of something much bigger.

It wasn't until a school work experience placement that nursing truly came into focus. At fifteen, I was placed in an aged care facility in Preston, Melbourne. Even now, I reflect on that experience with a sense of disbelief. On my very first day, I was asked to shower a male resident, something that would never be permitted for a student of that age today, and rightly so. But despite how confronting it was, that placement changed everything.

It was there that I met "John." He wasn't just another resident; he was a man who had lived many lives. Born in France, he had been a merchant marine and a member of the French Foreign Legion. He travelled extensively, worked in American hotels, and developed a deep appreciation for food and wine. He spoke of studying philosophy, theology, gardening, and astrology in Montreal, and told stories of bootlegging alcohol during Prohibition. After immigrating to Australia, he became a landscape gardener, a chauffeur to the wealthy, and later taught advanced French at Melbourne University. He was also regarded as an authority on growing liliums.

At fifteen, I did not yet have the language to articulate it, but I understood something fundamental, every resident carried a story, and those stories mattered.

Not all of my early lessons were so reflective. I remember assisting a resident with her lunch. She had no teeth, so her meal consisted of mashed vegetables and minced meat. As I fed her, a piece of potato became lodged in her mouth. Unsure what to do, I asked a nursing aide for advice. "Just hook it out with your finger," she said. So I did. What I was not prepared for was her biting down. My finger was trapped, and no matter how I tried, I couldn't free it. The nurse I was working with calmly remarked, "She sometimes tries to gum your finger to death." It was my first real introduction to the unpredictability of care, and to the dark humour nurses often rely on to cope.

During that short placement, I was also exposed to death for the first time, three times. At fifteen, it was confronting and difficult to process. I remember going home and speaking with my mother, trying to make sense of what I had witnessed. She gently explained that death was part of nursing, something I would have to learn to accept. Then she asked a simple question: "Do you want to go back?" I said yes. That was the moment I chose nursing.

Not everyone believed I would succeed. In Year 11, my maths teacher told me I would not amount to anything after I raised concerns about disruptive behaviour in the classroom. I failed that year, unfortunately in a subject required for nursing entry. It was a setback that could have easily ended the journey before it had properly begun.

Instead, it became part of the determination that followed.

At the time, it was the final year of hospital-based nursing programs, and I was unsuccessful in gaining a place. Instead, I was accepted into a large metropolitan university in Melbourne. So, at eighteen years old, I began my formal training.

Three hundred students filled the lecture theatre on that first day, three hundred strangers, each pursuing the same goal. It wasn't until we were divided into smaller groups for practical sessions that connections began to form. Some of those friendships would last a lifetime.

In first year, we studied anatomy and physiology in depth. Our lecturer set the tone early, making it clear that we would be working with human body parts donated for medical science and that they were to be treated with respect and dignity at all times. The message was firm: failure to do so could result in expulsion. It was enough to ensure that we approached every session with a mixture of reverence and apprehension.

We examined bones, muscles, skin, eyes, and brain tissue. It was both fascinating and confronting, but nothing quite prepared us for the day we studied reproductive anatomy. We were directed to a series of buckets lined up along the benches. With a simple nod from the lecturer, we lifted the lids. Inside were preserved male reproductive organs. For a group of eighteen-year-olds, fresh out of school, it was a moment of collective shock, equal parts disbelief, embarrassment, and nervous laughter. It was confronting, surreal, and unforgettable.

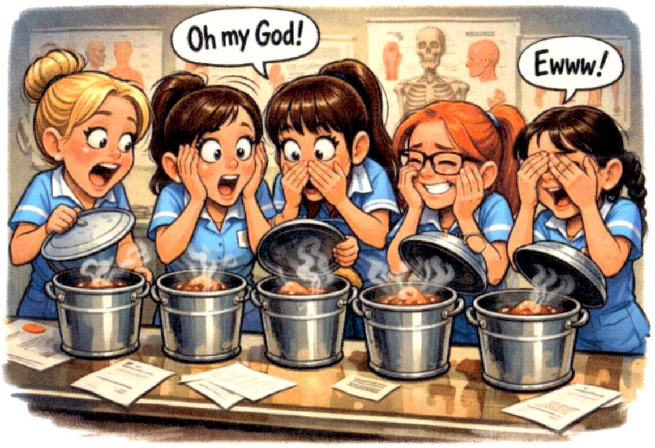

Another moment during a practical exam nearly ended in disaster. Moving between stations identifying anatomical structures, I examined a model head and lightly touched its cheek. The dentures fell straight into my hand. Time seemed to stop. My classmates gathered around as we frantically tried to reposition them, convinced we were about to be expelled. Somehow, we managed to fix the problem and move on, though not without a surge of panic.

Our first clinical placements were all in aged care facilities. We performed the basic tasks expected of student nurses, taking observations, assisting with personal hygiene, feeding residents, making beds, and emptying bedpans. Many residents were confined to their beds, while others were restrained in chairs. In one facility, the morning shower routine operated like a production line, with residents lined up and staff rotating through undressing, showering, and dressing. It was efficient, but it was also confronting, raising questions that I did not yet know how to answer.

During one placement, after reviewing an essay I had written, a clinical facilitator told me I would not make a “good” nurse. It was another moment that could have shaped my confidence differently but instead became part of the quiet resilience that was building.

By the end of first year, our cohort had halved, from 300 students to 150. Many left after their aged care placements, disillusioned by what they had seen. At the time, I shared that sentiment. I swore I would never work in aged care. I found aspects of it distressing, even confronting. I remember thinking that if these were my parents, I would never want them treated in that way. It is not lost on me that more than thirty years later, aged care would become my entire career.

Second year introduced more complexity, disease processes, ethics, research, chemistry, and physics, the latter being subjects I did not particularly enjoy. We also began preparing for acute care placements. Looking back, one of the most significant gaps in our education was dementia. We spent time studying the ageing process, but the depth and impact of dementia itself were barely explored. It left many of us underprepared for what we would later encounter in practice.

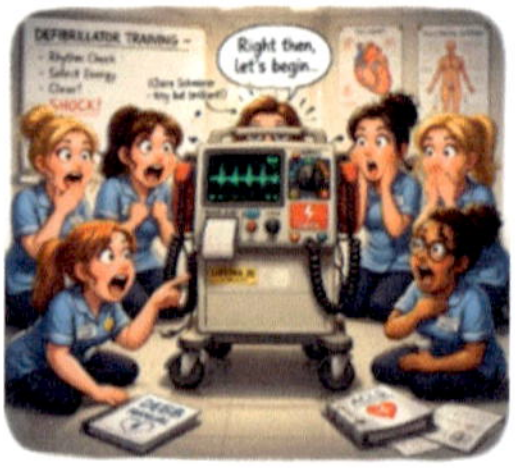

Before clinical placements, we practised essential skills, including the use of equipment such as defibrillators, large, wheeled machines with paddles and dials. It was during one of these sessions that I first encountered Claire Schmierer, although I had no idea at the time how influential she would later become in my life. What I do remember is that she was not very tall, and standing behind the defibrillator, she was almost entirely hidden.

Some practical sessions were more confronting than others. We were instructed to practise inserting nasogastric tubes, on each other. Unsurprisingly, none of us managed to get past the back of the throat.

Hospital placements in second year brought new responsibilities, and with them, inevitable mistakes. On one shift, I was asked to administer a gold injection. After preparing the medication, I went to change the needle and accidentally depressed the plunger, spraying the medication into the air. It was expensive, and the supervising nurse made it very clear that it was not a mistake to be repeated.

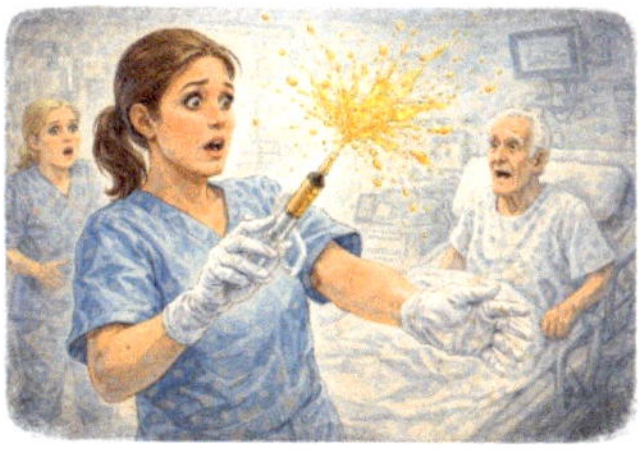

As university-trained students, we were not always welcomed by hospital-trained nurses. There was a clear divide, and at times, reluctance to teach us beyond basic tasks. However, even in those environments, the lessons we learned, whether intentional or not, were lasting.

During a debrief session, one student shared a story that stayed with me. They had found an elderly patient, presumed deceased, sitting in a chair. With assistance, they transferred the patient back to bed, only for the movement to stimulate a cardiac response. The nurse later advised them that next time, they should simply place a blanket over the patient and an oxygen mask on, without turning it on, so it appeared that something was being done. When this was shared with our ethics lecturer, the response was unexpected: “I wish you’d told me earlier, I could have included that in my book.” It was a moment that highlighted the gap between ethical theory and clinical reality.

Around this time, my grandmother became unwell and was admitted to hospital. During one visit, she told me her catheter had fallen out while she was on the toilet and had been reinserted while she was still sitting there. Even as a student, I knew this was not appropriate practice. She later developed a severe infection. It was a stark reminder that poor care was not abstract, it had real and personal consequences.

By third year, we were consolidating everything we had learned. During a women's health placement, one patient said to me, "A good nurse is born, not made, and I think you are one." It was the first time I had received such affirmation, and it stayed with me.

Over time, I came to understand that nursing in practice often differs from nursing in theory. Textbooks advised against crushing medications, yet in reality, we did so when patients could not swallow. Practical solutions often took precedence over ideal scenarios. Even something as simple as using Coca-Cola to unblock feeding tubes was not something you learned in a lecture.

We all took different paths after graduation. Some left the profession within a year, others excelled academically but struggled in practice, and some, like my friend Evelyn, built long and successful careers.

As for me, I completed my training in three years and have now spent over three decades in nursing, most of it in aged care, the very field I once said I would avoid. Along the way, I have presented at conferences, published articles, and built a career grounded in values I formed early on.

And through it all, some things have remained constant, particularly the friendships formed in those early years, friendships that, like the work itself, have endured the test of time.

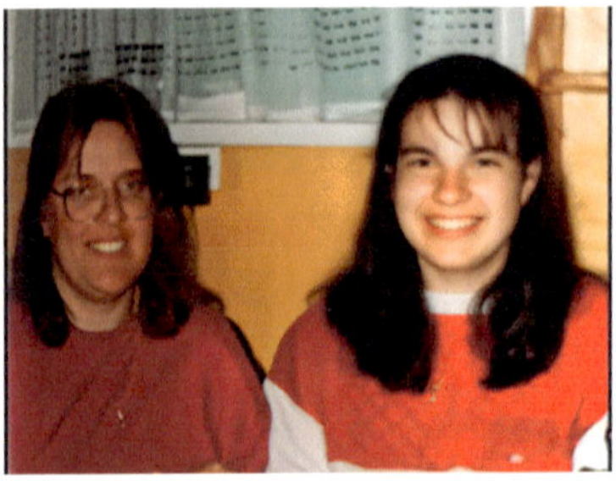

Evelyn & Susan (circa 1990)

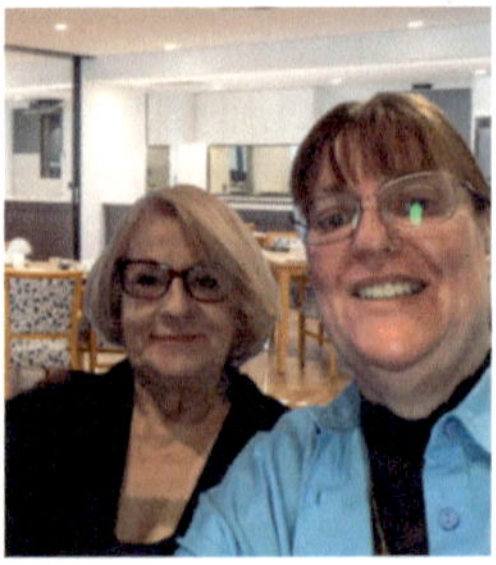

Claire & Susan (circa 2022)

Chapter 2
Graduate to Registered Nurse

Graduation was not the finish line, it was the beginning of a very different kind of learning. The structure and safety of university gave way to the realities of practice, where decisions carried weight and consequences were immediate.

Like many new nurses, I applied for a graduate program, hoping to remain close to home. Instead, I was offered a position in a small-to-mid-sized country hospital. I accepted, becoming the only "city" nurse in a group of ten graduates, most of whom were local. It was my first real experience of being both professionally and socially outside my comfort zone.

The hospital provided accommodation in what had once been the nurses' quarters. It had clearly seen better days. Bathrooms were shared and unisex, something that required a certain level of adjustment. The unspoken rule was simple: take everything with you when you shower, unless you were prepared to make an unintended appearance on your walk back to your room. After a couple of months, the novelty wore off. Add the constant presence of squatters, the exceptionally large huntsman spiders that seemed to have permanent residency, I decided it was time to find alternative accommodation.

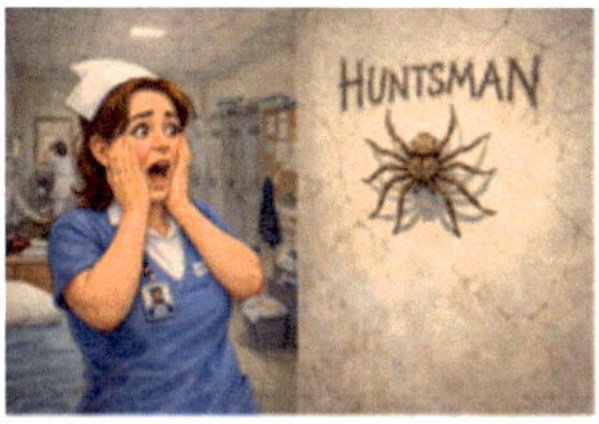

Working in a country hospital was far from the quiet, predictable experience I had imagined. During my time there, the facility went into lockdown due to an active shooter in the area, something I had never anticipated encountering so early in my career. It was a stark reminder that nursing does not exist in isolation from the world around it.

There were also smaller, more personal challenges that came with living independently in an unfamiliar place. One night after finishing a shift, my car refused to start. After calling roadside assistance and finally getting it running, I decided to drive around town to recharge the battery. It was close to midnight, the streets were empty, and inevitably, the car broke down again, this time in the middle of the road. A man appeared out of nowhere, pulling over to help. He casually mentioned he was out "driving his dog," which, at the time, seemed unusual, but I accepted the assistance. Once the car was restarted, I thanked him and drove home as quickly as possible, hoping that would be the end of the experience.

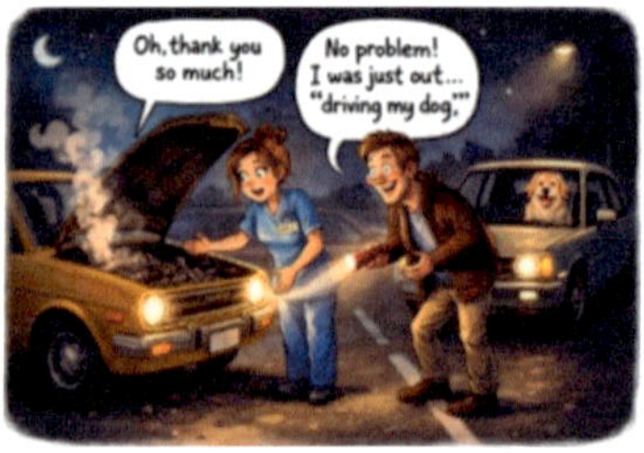

The graduate program rotated us through various wards, accompanied by written assignments and ongoing assessments. It didn't take long, however, to realise that the real learning did not come from textbooks or structured tasks. It happened on the floor, often in moments that were unexpected and confronting.

One such moment occurred when a doctor was taking arterial blood gases from an elderly patient. It is a delicate procedure, requiring precision and control. Under pressure, both literally and figuratively, the doctor applied too much force when transferring the sample into the vials. The needle disconnected from the syringe, and blood sprayed across the room. Including me. It soaked through my uniform, got under my glasses, and into my eyes. In the aftermath, I underwent months of hepatitis testing. It was a sharp and sobering reminder that no matter your role, mistakes do not discriminate in who they affect.

Other moments stayed with me for entirely different reasons. I remember caring for a teenage girl admitted following a pregnancy termination. What struck me most was not the procedure itself, but her response. As she recovered from the anaesthetic, her primary concern was that she didn't want to miss an episode of Neighbours. We turned on the television, and that was that. It was one of my earliest lessons in understanding that people process significant events in vastly different ways, and that our expectations do not always align with their reality.

Being the outsider within the graduate group was not easy. The other nurses had grown up together, studied together, and naturally gravitated towards one another outside of work. I was not part of that circle. Rather than resist it, I adapted. I arranged my shifts in blocks, often working ten consecutive days, so I could return to Melbourne during my time off. It became my way of maintaining connection to home while navigating a new environment.

Eventually, I returned to Melbourne permanently and joined a nursing agency. Initially, I appreciated the flexibility, but I was still searching for a role that offered stability and purpose. One particular shift ensured I would not stay in agency work for long.

I was assigned to a multi-storey aged care facility where the majority of residents did not speak English. That, in itself, was not the issue. The challenge was the staff. They spoke English but chose not to use it. Communication throughout the shift occurred almost entirely in their native language, leaving me isolated and unsupported. My assigned role quickly became limited to scraping leftover food from dinner plates. The medication round that followed was far more concerning, thirty residents, illegible handwriting, no one available to clarify orders, and no communication. It took two and a half hours to complete. By the end of both afternoon and evening rounds, I had spent nearly five hours administering medications. It was unsafe, unsustainable, and enough for me to decide I would not return.

Soon after, I secured a permanent position in a private rehabilitation unit, and it was here that my real education began.

For three years, I worked in closed head injury rehabilitation. The patients varied widely in age, but it was often the similarities, not the differences, that were most confronting. Some were children, the youngest just two years old. Others were my own age. That, perhaps, made it harder. These were not distant cases; they were reflections of how easily life could change for anyone, at any moment.

Many had arrived following preventable incidents, most commonly involving alcohol or drugs combined with driving. Occasionally, there were exceptions, a cow standing silently on a dark country road, or the reckless act of swapping seats in a moving vehicle, but more often than not, these were lives altered in an instant by a single decision. The consequences were immediate and irreversible.

Patients were often admitted within days of their injury. They arrived with tracheostomies, feeding tubes, and bodies sustained by machines while their futures remained uncertain. Some presented with severe pressure injuries. I recall one patient in particular who had wounds on both hips, each the size of a tennis ball and extending to the bone. We would work tirelessly to heal them, only for infection to set in. Each transfer back to hospital resulted in further deterioration, and each return meant starting the process again. It was a cycle that felt both relentless and, at times, avoidable.

Despite the emotional weight of the work, the staff found ways to cope. We had to. Humour became a form of release, a way of maintaining balance in an environment that was otherwise intense and unrelenting. We played practical jokes on one another, small, harmless moments that broke the tension. New staff might be asked to test a urine sample, only for a few drops of Mercurochrome to be added beforehand. The sudden appearance of "blood" would cause panic, quickly followed by laughter. It may have seemed inappropriate from the outside, but within that environment, it served a purpose.

Resources were often limited. There were rarely enough chairs at the nurses' station, so we would sit on the floor with files spread across our knees. I remember one afternoon charting in this way when a colleague approached, hiding a syringe of water behind his back. As he crouched beside me, he discreetly released the water beneath my paperwork. The reaction from the team was immediate, and my supposed "accident" became the focus of ongoing teasing for the remainder of the shift. In another setting, it may have been unacceptable. In ours, it was part of how we coped.

Most of us were in our twenties, navigating an environment filled with trauma and uncertainty. We relied heavily on each other. At times, once patients were settled, we would race wheelchairs down the corridors, brief, reckless moments that allowed us to release the tension that built up across each shift.

Within the team, I developed a reputation, one I carried with a mixture of humour and pride. Many male patients required condom drainage devices, and for reasons I could never fully explain, mine rarely failed. The nickname "Condom Queen" followed and, in that environment, it became a badge of reliability.

There were also moments that required a level of professionalism and advocacy beyond our years. One patient required a smaller-sized condom, yet his mother repeatedly replaced it with a larger one, convinced she knew best. It fell to me to address the situation, explaining clearly and respectfully why her actions were inappropriate. It was an early lesson in maintaining clinical boundaries, not only with patients, but with families.

The work could also be unpredictable and, at times, dangerous. As patients began to emerge from their injuries, confusion, agitation, and aggression were not uncommon. Safety was a constant consideration. There were occasions where multiple staff were required to safely complete a task, one to distract, another to support, and a third to act. While these approaches would not align with current practice standards, at the time they were often necessary, though never ideal.

I will never forget the day a patient struck a nurse across the face with a walking stick, breaking her nose. It was a stark reminder that while we were there to care, we were also vulnerable.

Of all the experiences during that time, one remains etched more deeply than the rest, the two-year-old boy.

He had sustained a severe brain injury and could not communicate, only whimper softly. The only way to comfort him was to hold him, to provide reassurance his body no longer understood how to process. So I did. As a young woman, newly married and thinking about my own future and family, it was almost unbearable. That experience stripped away any emotional distance I had tried to maintain.
Over those three years, I developed critical clinical skills, managing tracheostomies, complex wounds, catheter care, and PEG feeding. Most medications were crushed and administered through feeding tubes. These were technical competencies, but they were learned in an environment that demanded resilience just as much as skill.

Even within that seriousness, moments of levity remained. The unit manager and I would occasionally make bets on whether we could change a tracheostomy tube without triggering a cough, a near-impossible task. The stakes were simple: the loser bought a bottle of Chivas Regal. It was our way of bringing a sense of normality into highly clinical, high-pressure situations.

It was also during this time that my life outside of nursing continued to evolve. I met my husband, and we married. Life moved forward, even as work often felt heavy.

After three years, I transitioned into a geriatric rehabilitation unit, caring for post-surgical and medical patients. Not long after, I became pregnant with my first child. At seven and a half months, I stepped away from nursing and into motherhood. Over the following years, I had my second child and embraced a different kind of care, one that, in many ways, shaped me just as profoundly as my early years in nursing.

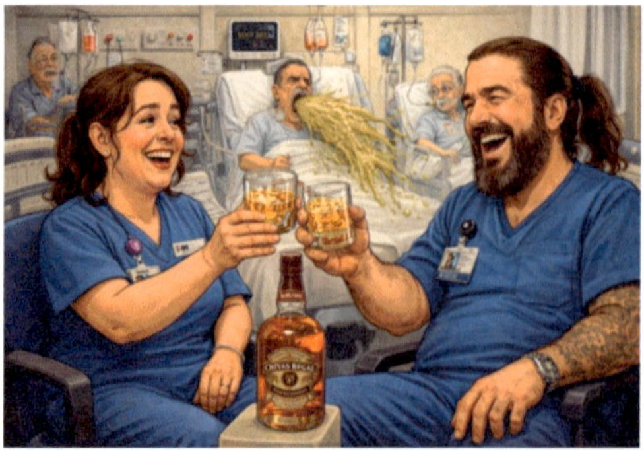

Chapter 3
Working Life After Children

I returned to the workforce in 1999. After several years away, I felt the need to both refresh and formalise my qualifications, so I enrolled at university to convert my Diploma of Nursing into a Bachelor's degree. Interestingly, I returned to the same institution where I had originally trained. Many of the lecturers were still there, including several professors who had taught me during my initial studies. In some ways, it felt like stepping back into a familiar space, but this time, I brought with me not only clinical experience, but life experience as well.

One lecture in particular highlighted how much perspective had shifted. Our ethics professor, who did not have children, spoke about witnessing a mother smack her toddler during a tantrum in a shopping centre and described it as abuse that should be reported. There was a noticeable change in the room. Many of us were now parents. While none of us condoned harm, we understood the reality of raising young children, the exhaustion, the unpredictability, and the moments where theory and lived experience do not align neatly. It was a clear example of how perspective evolves with experience.

During this time, I worked as an agency nurse, primarily in aged care. It was here that I became acutely aware of the stigma attached to the sector. In a class of twenty students, I was the only one working in aged care. The others were employed in areas such as emergency, paediatrics, and maternity. When we introduced ourselves, the reactions were subtle but unmistakable, raised eyebrows, polite nods, and underlying judgement.

The perception was clear: aged care was where nurses went when they were "winding down" or lacked clinical skill. I found that deeply confronting because what I was experiencing told a very different story.

In acute care, a typical shift might involve six patients, post-operative care, medications, observations, admissions, and discharges. Often, by mid-morning, I would be offering assistance to colleagues. In aged care, there was no such pause. A single shift involved managing more than thirty residents, medication rounds, wound care, documentation, staff supervision, liaising with doctors and allied health, responding to incidents, and supporting families.

The work was constant, complex, and demanding.

I was not bored, I was engaged, challenged, and responsible for coordinating care at a level I had not experienced elsewhere.

In acute care, I felt busy, In aged care, I felt useful.

The attitudes I encountered did not discourage me. Instead, they clarified something important. There was a clear disconnect within the profession, a gap between perception and reality, between what was valued and what truly required skill, judgement, and leadership.
Aged care sat on the wrong side of that divide.

Yet what I was experiencing on the floor told a different story entirely, one of complexity, responsibility, and purpose. It was a story I was already becoming deeply part of, whether the profession acknowledged it or not.

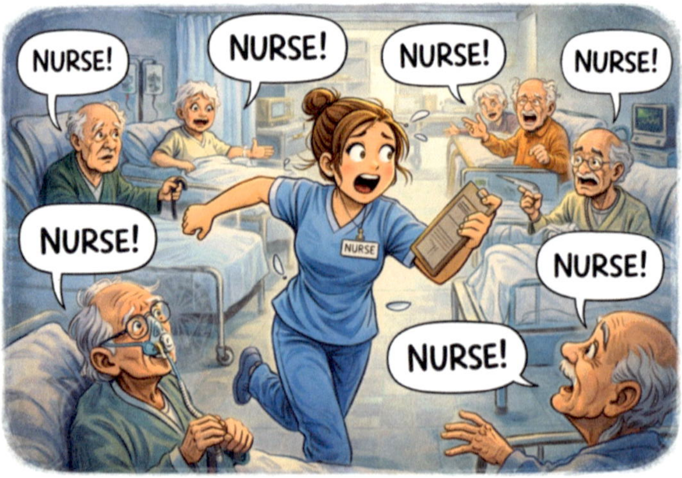

Chapter 4
Aged Care Journey

This was the beginning of my aged care journey.

Over the next seven years, I worked across two aged care homes, caring for between sixty and one hundred and ten residents at any given time. It was in these environments that I came to understand a fundamental truth, qualifying as a nurse does not make you a leader. Leadership is not something awarded with a certificate; it is learned through experience, tested in difficult moments, and often forged under pressure.

What became increasingly apparent to me was the absence of what are often referred to as "soft skills" among those stepping into leadership roles. Communication, conflict resolution, and the ability to guide and support others were rarely taught in any meaningful way, yet they were essential to maintaining both staff cohesion and resident care. These were skills I had to develop quickly, often in real time.

I remember one morning shift, barely thirty minutes in, when I heard raised voices in the corridor. It escalated rapidly into two staff members screaming at each other. Not arguing, screaming. Care had effectively stopped. I had no choice but to intervene, separating them, listening to both perspectives, and then restructuring the workload so the shift could continue safely. It was one of many moments where clinical knowledge alone was not enough. Leadership required presence, judgement, and the ability to restore order in the midst of chaos.

At university, we were taught that we might need to guide and educate doctors, that medicine could be procedural, while nursing often required a broader, more holistic view. What we were not taught was that sometimes this meant chasing a doctor into the car park, asking them to return and complete medication charts, and then negotiating when they refused. These were the realities no textbook prepared you for.

Returning to work after maternity leave provided what could only be described as a baptism by fire. My first shift back was in a secure dementia unit. There was one personal care worker and myself responsible for the entire area. I began a medication round in a shared room, approaching a resident gently, placing my hand on her arm and softly calling her name. Her response was immediate, a clenched fist connecting with my face. For a moment, all I could see were stars.

In the aftermath, I made an error and administered the wrong medications. The personal care worker later informed me, quite casually, that the resident was never woken that early. It would have been helpful to know. It was not the best return to practice, yet just two hours later, that same resident and I were dancing together to music. She had no recollection of what had occurred.

That was dementia care, unpredictable, confronting, and at times, unexpectedly joyful.

Many of my shifts were spent in a twenty-bed memory support unit, where one personal care worker and I were responsible for all residents. The routine was relentless. After handover, the personal care worker would begin showering and dressing residents while I commenced medication rounds. Once medications were completed, I would assist with showers, transfers, toileting, and meal preparation. Documentation was fitted in wherever possible, followed by more medications, more care, and ongoing coordination. That was on a "good" day.

At any point, the shift could be disrupted by behavioural incidents, falls, acute illness, or doctors' rounds. There was no downtime, only constant adjustment. On many occasions, I was the only registered nurse on site, responsible for medication administration for up to sixty residents, along with all clinical care, wound management, incident reporting, and staff support. The expectation was simple: everything would be completed, regardless of staffing levels or time constraints.

I stayed back countless hours after shifts to complete documentation and ensure safe handover. If those hours had been paid, I often joked, I would have retired a millionaire.

In one facility, it became increasingly common for me to be the sole registered nurse for one hundred and ten residents on an afternoon shift. I would begin a medication round, only to be called to another building, three hundred metres away, to administer insulin. I would walk down the hill, complete the injections, then walk back and resume the round. The system did not adapt, you did.

Despite the intensity, there were moments of humour that brought balance to the day. I remember a newly graduated personal care worker who had assisted a resident with dressing. Something didn't look quite right, but I couldn't immediately identify the issue. When I took the resident to her room, I discovered her bra had been put on backwards, with the cups at her back. It was a simple mistake, but one that stayed with me.

On another occasion, during a night shift, I pulled back a curtain and found a resident standing inches from my face, pale skin, white hair, white nightgown. I screamed loudly enough to wake half the facility. In that moment, she looked like a ghostly apparition.

There were also moments of unfiltered honesty that challenged assumptions. One resident's daughter had described her mother as "a real lady" who would never use inappropriate language. While assisting her in the shower, she calmly instructed me, "Don't forget to wash under the tits, dear." It was a reminder that people often defy the narratives others create for them.

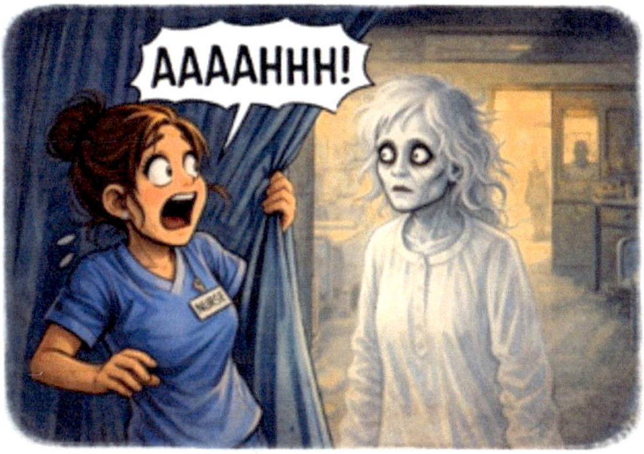

Continence aids were often held in place by knitted mesh underpants. During a medication round one morning, I rounded a corner with the medication trolley with my head down. When I raised it, the sight before

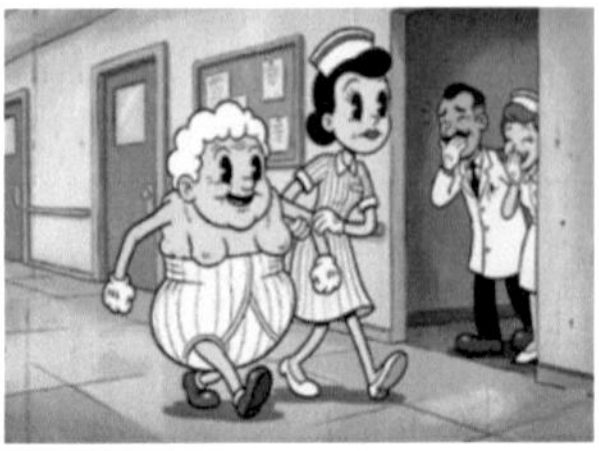

me stayed with me all my life. There was a small in stature female resident with only the continence aid and the underpants pulled up to her armpits with her breasts tucked in. She was well endowed and they were hanging down as they do when we ladies got older, to her belly button.

Aggression was, unfortunately, a regular part of the role. While it should never be considered acceptable, it was a reality when working with residents living with dementia. Over time, I was bitten, punched, kicked, spat on, placed in a headlock, and even punched in the stomach while pregnant with my third child.

One night shift stands out clearly. After lowering the volume on a resident's television, they became agitated. When I returned to check on them, they placed me in a headlock. With assistance, we guided them back to their room, but as we attempted to leave, they lunged again. I instinctively grabbed their wrists to protect myself and was bitten on the arm, leaving a full set of teeth marks. The resident had no PRN medication charted, so I contacted a locum doctor. He arrived, looked at my arm, laughed, and suggested he had a WWE wrestling video in his car that might help me "learn a few moves."

The following morning, when I reported the incident, management's response was simple: "It was your fault. You shouldn't have turned the TV down." That moment stayed with me, not because of the injury, but because of what it revealed about how staff safety was valued.

Not all memories were chaotic; some were deeply unsettling in a different way. On one night shift, a resident who was non-weight bearing and unable to mobilise independently passed away. At 2 a.m., he had been checked and was comfortable in bed. At 4 a.m., he was found deceased, on his knees, leaning forward against the bed, as though in prayer. It was assumed he had suffered an acute event causing a sudden spasm, but the image has never left me.

It was also during this time that I began to observe management practices more closely, and not always positively. I witnessed decisions that prioritised efficiency over dignity. On one occasion, after a resident had passed away, their body was moved into another resident's room so the bed could be filled immediately with a new admission. That moment defined something for me. If I ever moved into management, I would not lead that way.

After one manager left due to a conflict of interest, I was asked to assist with administrative duties. By then, I had just had my third child. The interim manager, Claire Schmierer, who had once been my university lecturer, allowed me to bring my six-week-old baby to work. For two to three months, my son came with me each day. When he cried, I would answer phones one-handed while feeding him. Often, I would return to find him missing from his pram, only to discover he had been carried off by residents, passed gently from one set of arms to another. He became, quite unintentionally, part of the community.

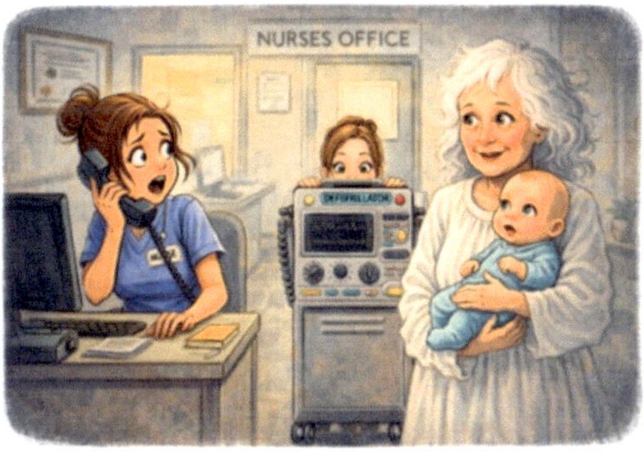

It was also during this time that I had my first real experience with computers. Reports needed to be emailed to head office, something I had never done before. It took me most of a day to work out how to attach documents and send them. When I proudly shared this achievement at home, my eight-year-old son casually informed me, "You should have called me, Mum, we learned that at school." It was a humbling moment.

Working in an Italian-focused facility also expanded my education in unexpected ways. Despite having studied Italian briefly in high school, it was here that I became fluent, particularly in colourful language. One resident would greet me daily with "Puttana," ensuring my vocabulary developed rapidly, whether I wanted it to or not.
Even interactions with ambulance crews became part of the rhythm of the job. After one resident refused hospital transfer during an evening shift, the same crew returned the following morning for a serious head injury. Seeing me on the floor, covered in blood and holding a compression dressing, they joked, "So... is it a real call this time?" This time, it was.

These years shaped me in ways no formal education ever could. They taught me resilience, adaptability, and the reality of leadership in its rawest form. They also reinforced something that would stay with me throughout my career, aged care is often underestimated, yet it demands a level of skill, judgement, and emotional strength that is unlike any other area of nursing.

And I was only just beginning to understand it.

Chapter 5
Stepping Up: Management
(You'll Only Do This Once)

My final year at one of these facilities marked the beginning of my transition into management. I was appointed Deputy Director of Nursing, a role I held for twelve months before moving on. It was my first real step away from purely clinical work and into a position where responsibility extended beyond individual residents to the systems and staff supporting their care.

In that role, I oversaw approximately forty residents, supported primarily by enrolled nurses. Around this time, the workforce within aged care began to shift noticeably. Shortages of registered and enrolled nurses became increasingly common, and personal care workers began to fill the gaps. Alongside this shift came the rise of inconsistent training providers, producing a workforce with varying levels of skill and understanding. Over time, training evolved to allow personal care workers to administer medications from dose administration aids, further blurring the boundaries between roles and responsibilities.

My next position was as a unit manager in a sixty-bed facility, comprising forty-five low-care residents and a fifteen-bed high-care unit. It was here that I encountered some of the more confronting realities of aged care, resident aggression, poor management practices, and systemic failures that challenged both my professional confidence and personal resilience.

One incident in particular has never left me.

At the time, I worked Monday to Friday, 7 am to 3 pm, as the registered nurse on site. After hours, care was handed over to enrolled nurses and personal care staff. A ninety-two-year-old female resident, living with macular degeneration, dementia, and metastatic breast cancer, suffered a fall resulting in a fractured neck of femur. She was transferred to a large metropolitan hospital, where she underwent surgical repair and required multiple blood transfusions.

Soon after, her family contacted me. They were distressed and believed she was in significant pain. They asked me to advocate for her while she remained in acute care. When I spoke with hospital staff, I was told her vocalisations, her moaning and groaning, were attributed to dementia rather than pain. They had contacted the facility and spoken with a staff member who reassured them that this behaviour was "normal" for her. It was later established that the person they spoke to was the owner/manager, who was both a personal care worker and a family acquaintance of the resident.

But it wasn't normal.

Further discussions led to a decision to proceed with prophylactic surgery on her other hip. When she was eventually discharged back to the facility on Thursday afternoon, she arrived in obvious, uncontrolled pain. Her pain management was inadequate, limited to a patch and intermittent subcutaneous morphine injections.

I stayed until midnight that evening, trying to stabilise her pain. At 6 am the following morning, I returned after receiving a call from the enrolled nurse, her pain had worsened, and the nurse on duty was unable to administer injections. That day, I arranged an urgent referral to palliative care. By 5 pm, a syringe driver had been commenced. By 7 pm, she finally appeared to be resting comfortably.

At 7 am the following morning, I received the call, she had passed away.

Despite the family expressing nothing but gratitude for the care I provided in her final days, the experience stayed with me. It left a lingering sense of failure, one that colleagues later reassured me did not belong to me, but to a system that had failed her long before she returned to my care. Even so, that knowledge never fully lifted the weight of it.

Her death became a defining moment in my career, a line I drew within myself. A quiet but resolute commitment that I would never again allow a resident under my care to experience that level of unmanaged suffering without exhausting every possible avenue for dignity and comfort.
Not all challenges during this time were clinical.

There were occasions where I found myself having to justify clinical decisions to a manager with no formal qualifications, someone whose authority came not from knowledge or experience, but from ownership. Medication management was frequently questioned, often without understanding, creating an environment where clinical judgement was undermined.

The breaking point came when I witnessed this same manager berating a resident for being incontinent. She stood over the woman, wagging her finger, raising her voice, and telling her she was "never to pee on the floor again." This was in a facility where residents were not permitted commode chairs in their rooms and were expected to mobilise to the bathroom regardless of their physical limitations. That moment crystallised everything and I knew I had to leave.

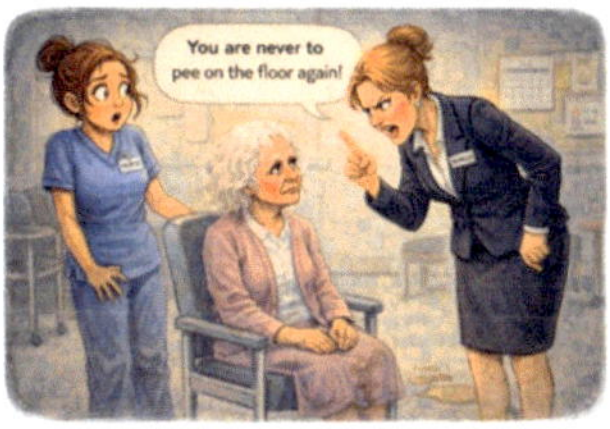

From there, I moved into my first true leadership role, managing a hostel. It was during this time that my perspective on aged care began to shift. I undertook specialised training in Advanced Care Planning and became an associate in the Eden Philosophy, an approach that challenged traditional models of care and reframed how we viewed ageing, dignity, and quality of life.

Advanced Care Planning quickly became a priority. We organised a meeting with local general practitioners to introduce and embed it within the facility. I was asked to speak, and I shared the story of the resident whose painful death had remained with me, how the absence of a clear, documented plan had contributed to unnecessary suffering, and how deeply it had affected me both professionally and personally.

Afterwards, several doctors approached me. They told me it was not my failure, that the system had let her down. I appreciated their reassurance, but it did not erase the sense of responsibility I carried.

What the Eden Philosophy offered, however, was something different. It reframed care entirely, not as a series of tasks or clinical interventions, but as a human experience that required connection, meaning, and dignity at every stage.

The Eden Philosophy

The Eden Philosophy teaches that the greatest suffering in ageing does not come from disease, but from three plagues: loneliness, helplessness, and boredom. Its principles challenge us to create environments where life continues to be meaningful, connected, and human.

My Eden journey began in 2007, and it was nothing short of transformative.
The training was immersive and confronting in the best possible way. It asked us not just to change systems, but to change ourselves, to reflect, to feel, and to reconnect with the humanity at the heart of care.

I became an Eden Philosophy Associate. The Eden Philosophy suggests that by addressing the three "plagues" of ageing, loneliness, helplessness, and boredom, we can change and improve the final years of our elders" journey.

When I returned to the facility, I wanted to test what I had learned. I brought in a bunch of carnations and handed them to the receptionist, asking her to give them out to residents "just because." She hesitated, confused, but she did it. When she returned, her face was lit with a smile that stayed with her for the rest of the day.

Then came the marshmallows. I handed a packet to another receptionist and told her to start a marshmallow fight in the lounge. When I checked in later, I found her wearing gloves and a kitchen hat, carefully handing out marshmallows one at a time on toothpicks.

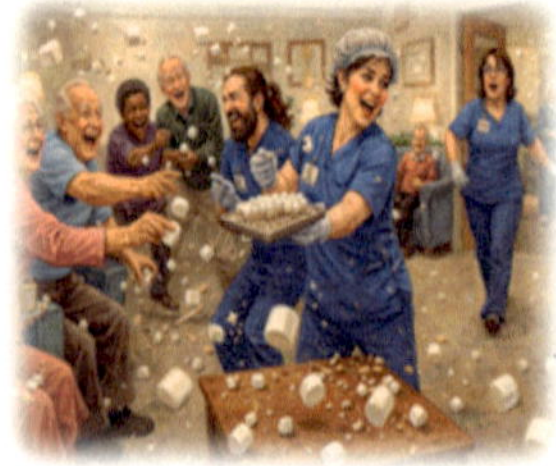

"What are you doing?" I asked.
"Giving out the marshmallows," she replied.
Laughing, I said, "No, this is a marshmallow fight. Throw them."
She looked horrified. "What about infection control?"

And in that moment, it became painfully clear, What had we done? We had regulated the joy out of living. We had replaced spontaneity with policy, connection with compliance, and humanity with risk management. As leaders, we set the tone. If we cannot embrace what matters, if we cannot model compassion, spontaneity, and courage, then we cannot expect it from those around us.

Change does not start with policy. It starts with us.

"Well-being is a much larger idea than either quality of life or customer satisfaction. It is based on a holistic understanding of human needs and capacities. Well-being is elusive, highly subjective, and the most valuable of all human possessions."
Dr Bill Thomas, from A life Worth Living.

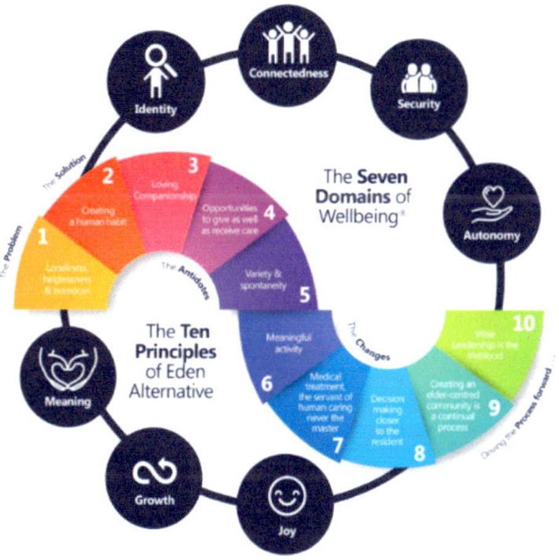

The **Eden Alternative Domains of Well-Being®** are 7 fundamental aspects of personhood that underpin the core of our Framework. They are the outcomes care partners achieve when they put the Ten Principles of the Eden Alternative into action. – **https://edeninoznz.com.au**

Chapter 6
Navigating Staff Culture
(The Hardest Part of the Job)

By 2007, mandatory reporting had been legislated. On paper, it was a necessary and overdue reform designed to protect the most vulnerable. In practice, it introduced a level of complexity that few were truly prepared for. Over the following years, I managed two serious reportable incidents involving allegations of inappropriate touching by staff. Both cases were ultimately unsubstantiated as there was no evidence to support the claims. However, the absence of evidence did little to protect those involved. Reputations were damaged, trust was eroded, and the emotional toll on everyone including staff, families, and myself was significant. These situations required a careful balance between protecting residents and ensuring fairness for staff, a balance that is far more difficult to achieve in reality than policy would suggest.

As my career progressed, I moved through various leadership roles, from Care Coordinator to Facility Manager and eventually Regional Quality Manager across multiple sites. While there were many rewarding moments, the most challenging experiences were almost always linked to staff behaviour rather than systems or processes. These situations not only tested my professional capabilities but also my resilience, values, and ability to lead under pressure.

One such incident involved a serious medication error. Two staff members failed to follow correct procedures when administering Schedule 8 analgesia. The medication was neither signed out correctly nor documented on the medication chart, resulting in a resident being overdosed. I discovered the issue during a routine medication audit and immediately went to assess the resident, who was unresponsive. The seriousness of the situation was undeniable. Later, at handover, I addressed the incident with the staff involved, including a newly graduated enrolled nurse. Despite the gravity of what had occurred, her response was defensive rather than reflective. She simply stated, "we work hard, you know." In that moment, it became clear that while knowledge and skills can be developed, accountability and professional insight are far more difficult to instil.

In another role, I encountered a long-term nurse who initially appeared to be an asset to the organisation. However, it soon became evident that her practice was deeply flawed. A complaint triggered an investigation, revealing that she had failed to implement appropriate treatment for an acutely unwell resident, resulting in hospitalisation. Further concerns emerged, including intimidating behaviour towards residents and dismissive interactions with families. In one instance, she discarded a written complaint in front of a family member because it implicated her own practice. When performance management was initiated, rather than acknowledging the issues, she responded with counter-allegations of bullying and racial discrimination. This created a highly stressful environment, both professionally and personally, reinforcing just how complex and emotionally taxing leadership can be when accountability is absent.

Despite these challenges, there were moments that reminded me why I remained committed to aged care. One of the most memorable was the adoption of Snowy, a retired racing greyhound who had suffered a broken hip. Snowy quickly became part of the home, often resting on the couch outside my office. He had a gentle way of engaging with people, slowly approaching visitors and leaning into them for affection. His presence had a profound impact on residents, particularly one woman with advanced dementia who would sit quietly while Snowy rested his head on her lap. She would stroke him as she drifted off to sleep. On one occasion, her husband arrived and was visibly surprised, telling me she had never liked dogs prior to entering care. Yet here she was, calm and content. Snowy brought a level of comfort and connection that no clinical intervention could replicate. When I eventually left the facility, I took Snowy home, as the incoming manager did not support having animals on site.

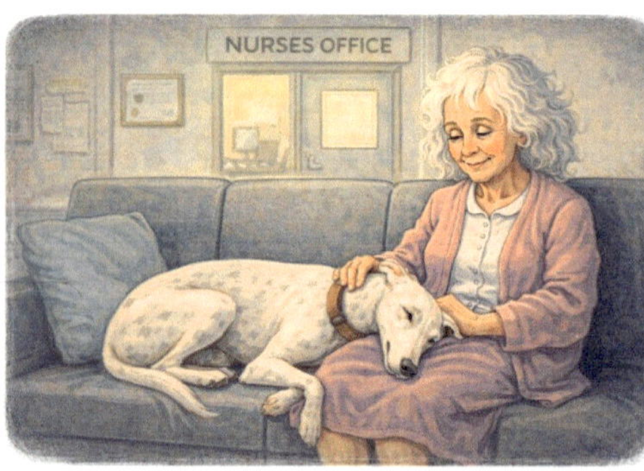

Not all situations were so gentle. There were times when I was required to manage incidents far outside the scope of any formal training. On one occasion, a family member became aggressive during a visit and struck a resident. I was called to intervene and found the individual visibly agitated, pacing and highly distressed. I calmly requested that he leave and escorted him out of the building via the fire stairs. Afterwards, staff discovered an imitation handgun in the resident's room, which had been used in the assault. Further investigation revealed that this individual had a history of serious violent offending. It was a confronting experience and one that highlighted the unpredictable nature of the role. That evening, I went home and attempted to process what had occurred, aware that these were situations no training could fully prepare you for.

There were also moments of unexpected humour that helped balance the intensity of the role. On one occasion, I heard a "Code Pink" announced over the PA system and immediately assumed it was a clinical emergency. I rushed down several flights of stairs, only to be met with laughter from administration staff who informed me that it referred to a "cute fireman" arriving to check the alarms. It was a reminder that not every urgent call required the same level of response, and sometimes perspective was everything.

Person-centred care remained central to my practice. One resident expressed a dying wish to marry her partner. While a formal wedding was not feasible, we created a meaningful alternative. We organised a commitment ceremony within the facility, complete with rings, a wedding cake, and a car ride around the block. I officiated the ceremony, and residents and staff came together to celebrate the occasion. The resident passed away not long after, but she did so having experienced a moment of joy and fulfilment. It reinforced for me that care is not only about managing clinical needs, but about honouring what matters most to the individual.

Supporting and mentoring staff became an equally important part of my role, although it is often overlooked in management. I was asked to mentor a newly graduated registered nurse completing his graduate year. He was a pleasure to work with, thoughtful, committed, and honest about his doubts regarding his career path. Despite these uncertainties, he persevered. Over time, he not only continued working in aged care but also expanded his contribution to the health industry through additional ventures. He remains someone I deeply respect, and I am proud to call him both a colleague and a friend. Experiences like this reinforced that leadership is not just about managing performance, but about investing in people and helping them find their place within the profession.

There were also lighter moments that brought teams together and reminded us not to take ourselves too seriously. On one occasion, for my birthday, the staff organised a surprise. One of the male staff members appeared in an off-the-shoulder mini dress and six-inch stilettos, singing happy birthday. I remember joking that I was jealous, he had better legs than I did. The residents laughed for hours, and for a moment, the usual pressures of the environment faded. These moments of shared humour and humanity were just as important as any clinical intervention.
Throughout my career, I had witnessed poor leadership from those in management positions, and I made a conscious decision that I would lead differently. However, maintaining that commitment was not always easy. I was asked on multiple occasions to act in ways that conflicted with my values, including terminating staff for reasons unrelated to performance, overlooking poor practice, or remaining silent in the face of misconduct. I refused to compromise, even when it meant walking away from roles. In one facility, I resigned after six weeks due to unsafe and unethical practices, including inappropriate medication administration and a culture that prioritised appearances over actual care.

In another setting, I encountered resistance to evidence-based practice when implementing wound care recommendations from a specialist. Despite initial opposition from long-standing staff, the changes led to significant improvement and eventual healing of a chronic wound. This experience reinforced the importance of challenging outdated practices and advocating for better outcomes, even when it is uncomfortable to do so.

Leadership, I came to understand, is not about authority or position. It is about influence, consistency, and the willingness to act. In one instance, I responded to a resident who had become unwell in a common area. While directing staff, I also began assisting with cleaning. A staff member expressed shock, stating that as the manager, I should not be doing such tasks. However, I believed then, as I do now, that leadership requires visibility and participation. The reaction from staff highlighted how uncommon this approach had become, and perhaps why culture within some facilities had deteriorated.

Over time, I continued to build my knowledge through further education in areas such as palliative care, dementia management, medication safety, and training. However, the most valuable lessons did not come from formal study. They came from experience, from mentorship, and from the people I worked alongside. Mentors like Claire demonstrated what strong, values-based leadership looked like, and in turn, influenced the way I supported others, including new graduates entering the profession.

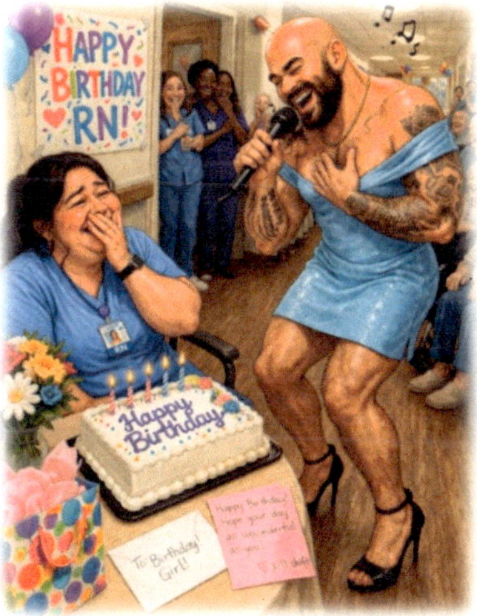

Ultimately, staff culture is shaped by leadership. Poor leadership creates environments where poor practice is tolerated, accountability is avoided, and residents suffer as a result. Conversely, strong leadership fosters respect, responsibility, and quality care. Throughout my career, I have remained guided by a simple principle: never compromise on the standard of care or the values that underpin it. Because at the end of the day, culture is not dictated by policy, it is defined by what leaders are willing to accept, challenge, and change.

Chapter 7
Shaping My Leadership Style

From 2013 to 2020, my career began to extend beyond the immediate environment of individual facilities and into the broader aged care sector. During this time, I had the opportunity to contribute articles to industry publications and attend both state and national conferences. One of my articles on leadership was published in LASA Fusion, and in 2017 I delivered a digital presentation at the LASA National Conference titled "Dementia 2020 and Beyond". These experiences allowed me to step back from the operational pressures of the floor and begin to see the industry through a wider lens, reinforcing that leadership is not confined to a single workplace but has the potential to influence thinking and practice across the sector.

The conferences themselves were as much about connection as they were about learning. One of my earliest experiences was attending a conference dinner themed Rocky Horror Picture Show. I remember arriving with the quiet assumption that most people would take a conservative approach to dressing up. Instead, I walked into a room filled with senior leaders and CEOs fully embracing the theme, fishnet stockings, high heels, gold shorts, and more than a few Frank-N-Furters. It was unexpected, but it revealed something important, behind the titles and responsibilities were people capable of humour, vulnerability, and genuine connection. That insight stayed with me.

At another conference, the theme was circus. I attended with a group of managers, our general manager dressed as the ringmaster while the rest of us committed to being clowns, complete with red noses and brightly coloured wigs. The venue was within walking distance, so we made our way there and back on foot. The reactions from people passing by as we danced our way to the venue were unforgettable, ranging from amusement to outright confusion. While light-hearted, these moments reinforced an important aspect of leadership, that authenticity and the ability to connect with others, even through humour, are just as important as technical competence.

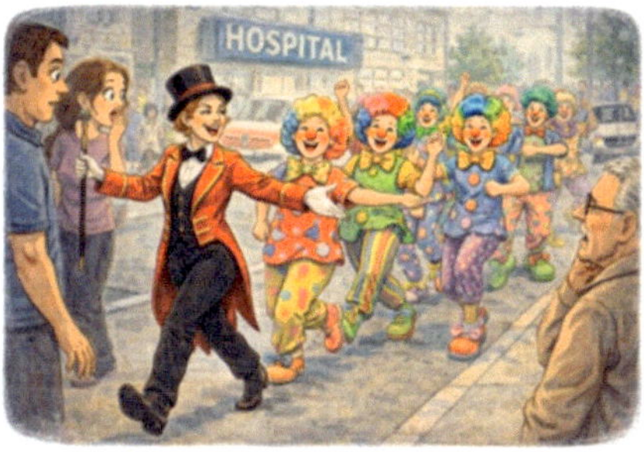

My next role saw me overseeing more than twelve facilities as a Quality and Education Manager, a position that shifted my perspective significantly. I was no longer immersed solely in the day-to-day clinical work but instead responsible for observing, guiding, and improving practice across multiple sites. During this time, I completed further training in Managing Actual and Potential Aggression, which enabled me to educate staff as part of a "train the trainer" model. It was a valuable skill set, but the greatest learning came not from the course itself, but from what I observed in practice.

Stepping away from the floor allowed me to see patterns that had previously been less visible. The gaps in fundamental nursing practice were more significant than I had anticipated. Communication, both verbal and written, was often lacking clarity and consistency. Assessments were incomplete, care plans were not followed through, pathology results were not always reviewed, and handovers sometimes failed to convey critical information. Alongside this, there were instances of unprofessional behaviour that raised concerns not only about individual practice but about the broader culture within some teams.

What I encountered repeatedly was the phrase, “we don’t have time.” It became a common explanation for incomplete tasks and missed responsibilities. However, this reasoning did not sit comfortably with me. Throughout my own clinical career, I had always worked until my responsibilities were complete, understanding that unfinished work often translated directly into compromised care. The idea that essential tasks could be left undone without a sense of accountability was deeply unsettling. Over time, it became clear that the issue was not always a lack of time, but rather a combination of prioritisation, systems, and professional ownership.

This was particularly evident during a medication audit of a Dangerous Drug cupboard. Staff had explained that completing the medication count could take over an hour, which initially suggested a workload issue. However, when I examined the cupboard, the underlying problem became clear. Following regulatory changes requiring codeine-based medications to be stored as controlled drugs, stock levels had not been adjusted accordingly. One resident, who only required occasional doses of Panadeine Forte, had accumulated more than one thousand tablets. As each tablet had to be counted individually, the process had become unnecessarily time-consuming. What had been perceived as a staffing or time issue was a lack of review and critical oversight. A simple adjustment to ordering practices could have resolved the problem entirely.

Another situation that significantly shaped my leadership approach involved a resident who consistently became physically resistive during personal care. Staff expressed frustration and confusion, unable to understand why routine hygiene tasks triggered such strong reactions. When I worked through the situation with the team, I began by exploring the resident’s background. He was a Jewish man who had migrated to Australia after World War II. I asked staff how they approached him when assisting with showers. Their responses were consistent, typically along the lines of “it’s time for your shower” which brought back memories of war atrocities he had faced.

It was at this point that a deeper understanding was required. Many of the staff were younger and had limited awareness of the historical trauma experienced by Jewish people during the war. I explained that the language being used could act as a trigger, linked to fear, persecution, and the experiences associated with concentration camps. To the resident, those words did not represent care, they represented threat and loss of control. Once the team understood this, we changed our approach, adjusting our language and ensuring this was clearly documented in the care plan. The impact was immediate, with a noticeable reduction in distress and resistance. It reinforced a fundamental truth: behaviour is often a form of communication, and without understanding the person behind it, care can unintentionally cause harm.

Experiences like these reshaped how I viewed leadership. It became less about enforcing compliance and more about fostering understanding. Policies and procedures provide structure, but they do not replace critical thinking or empathy. Effective leadership requires creating an environment where staff feel supported to question, reflect, and improve, rather than simply follow instructions without context.

Over time, I came to recognise that many of the challenges within aged care are not solely the result of limited resources, but of gaps in knowledge, communication, and accountability. Addressing these issues requires more than systems, it requires leadership that is present, engaged, and willing to guide others through complexity rather than avoid it.

These years played a significant role in shaping my leadership style. They reinforced that leadership is not defined by position or authority, but by influence, consistency, and the ability to bring clarity where there is confusion. It is about recognising that behind every task, every behaviour, and every challenge, there is a deeper story, one that has the potential to change outcomes entirely.

Chapter 8
The COVID-19 Pandemic

It was during my time with this organisation that the COVID-19 pandemic emerged, an experience I hope never to repeat. What began as a global health crisis quickly became something far more complex within aged care. Alongside the virus itself came fear, misinformation, and intense media scrutiny, which often translated into public judgment directed at those working within residential facilities. While there were undoubtedly cases where outbreaks were mismanaged, there were just as many where staff did everything humanly possible under extraordinarily difficult circumstances.

The reality on the ground was far removed from the narratives often portrayed. Staff were not only managing infection control but also the emotional distress of residents and families. Restrictions on visitation, though necessary, were devastating. Families, unable to see their loved ones, would gather outside facilities, distressed and often angry. There were times we had to employ security guards to manage the situation, as staff were subjected to verbal abuse simply for enforcing public health directives. It was a stark reminder that in times of crisis, those on the frontline can become the focus of frustration, regardless of their intentions or efforts.

Managing an outbreak of this magnitude required a level of endurance I had never previously experienced. For a period of three months, I underwent nasal swabbing every second day. Staffing shortages became critical as employees either contracted the virus or were too fearful to attend work. Those who remained had to take on multiple roles, becoming, quite literally, everything the facility needed them to be.

A typical day during this time bore little resemblance to anything I had known before. My shifts often began at 7:00 am and extended well into the evening, sometimes finishing at 11:00 pm, and this continued for twenty-three consecutive days without a break. The responsibilities were relentless and varied from managing staff, providing education, administering medications, delivering hands-on clinical care, restocking PPE stations, assisting with laundry and kitchen duties to more formal requirements of attending daily meetings with both the Department of Health and head office to report on outbreak status.

The physical toll was equally significant. Working continuously in full PPE led to rapid weight loss, I lost six kilograms in six weeks. Masks and goggles caused skin irritation, bruising across the bridge of the nose, and blisters behind the ears. Fatigue became a constant companion, but there was little time to acknowledge it. The focus remained on keeping residents safe.

What made this period particularly challenging was the disconnect between frontline realities and organisational oversight. Daily head office meetings were intended to demonstrate support, yet often consisted of staff working from home, offering words of appreciation from a distance. While those sentiments were no doubt genuine, they did not fully capture or alleviate the intensity of what was happening within the facilities. The difference between experiencing the outbreak and observing it remotely was profound.

One incident during this time remains particularly difficult to reflect on. A resident was transferred to hospital for a non-COVID-related acute condition. Shortly after, the resident was returned to the facility. When I questioned the ambulance staff, I was informed that the resident had not even been taken inside the hospital. Instead, medical personnel had assessed the situation from the open doors of the ambulance, determined that the resident appeared stable, and instructed that they be returned.

It was one of the few times in my career that I cried at work.

The lack of dignity, care, and respect shown to an elderly and vulnerable individual was confronting. Despite having no support from the acute health service, our already exhausted team managed the resident's care within the facility. With careful monitoring and appropriate interventions, the resident recovered. While the outcome was positive, the circumstances surrounding it highlighted the broader challenges faced by aged care during the pandemic.

Amidst the intensity, there were brief moments that provided relief. On one occasion, we received a delivery of bright orange hazmat suits. At that time, we were able to allow a small number of residents out of their rooms to sit in the lounge. In an attempt to lift spirits, I gathered several members of the senior team, and we put on the suits. Together, we performed a light-hearted sing-along to "Oompa Loompa" from Charlie and the Chocolate Factory. For a short time, laughter replaced anxiety. It was a simple gesture, but one that reminded us of the importance of maintaining human connection, even in the most challenging circumstances. I believe that moment made its way onto the nightly news as we had many reporters outside the facility.

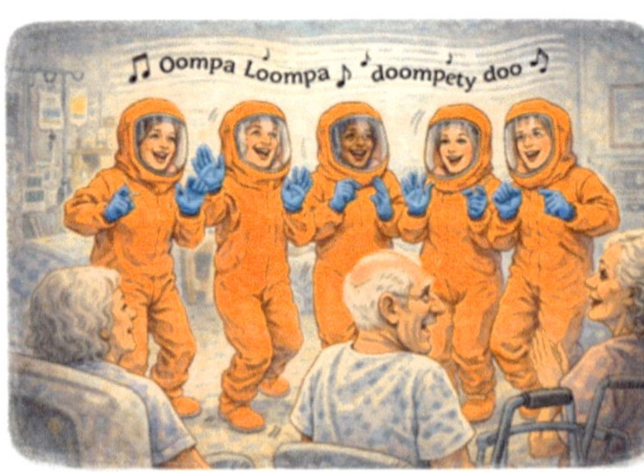

Throughout this period, my role as an internal auditor and quality manager also continued to shape my perspective. I observed how staff carried out their duties under pressure, and it reinforced a question that had been building for some time. The phrase "we don't have time" was still commonly used to explain incomplete tasks, yet I could not reconcile this with what I knew to be achievable.

Having spent many years working "on the floor", I understood the demands of the role. A shift involved administering medications, completing clinical care such as observations and wound management, liaising with allied health professionals and doctors, documenting care, updating assessments and care plans, and providing a comprehensive handover. If time allowed, you helped with personal care tasks to support the team. These expectations had not fundamentally changed. What had changed, however, was the perception of what was manageable.

I found myself questioning how responsibilities that had once been considered standard practice had come to be viewed as excessive. Many of the nurses expressing these concerns were younger and physically capable, yet the sense of ownership and completion that had once defined the role seemed to be diminishing.

The pandemic did not create these issues, but it exposed them.

It revealed both the strength and the fragility of the system, highlighting the dedication of those who stepped up, while also bringing into focus the areas where accountability, resilience, and professional standards needed to be reinforced.

Looking back, COVID-19 was more than a health crisis. It was a defining period that tested leadership, systems, and individuals in ways few could have anticipated. It reinforced the importance of adaptability, presence, and leading from the front, while also reminding me that even in the most difficult times, moments of humanity can make all the difference, no matter how small.

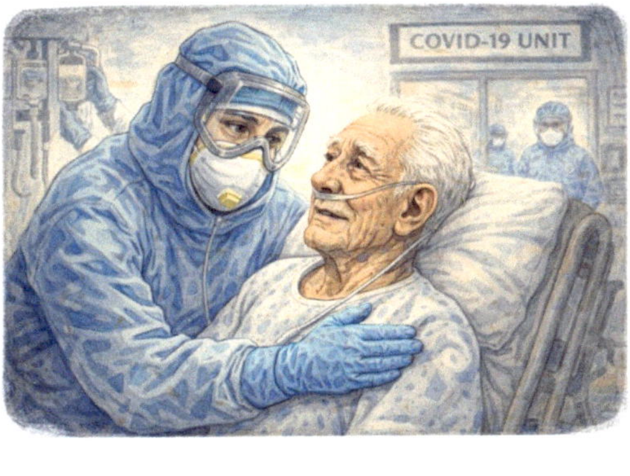

Chapter 9
Edgarley CEO

By the end of 2020, after the initial wave of COVID-19, I reached a turning point in my career. For many years, I had worked within large national organisations where decisions were often made far removed from the realities of the floor. Increasingly, I found myself implementing directives that I did not always agree with, decisions that had drifted away from what mattered most: the resident.

I wanted something different.

I wanted to be in a position where I could make decisions, not just carry them out. Throughout my career, my focus had always been the same, resident first, always. Financial drivers had never been my motivation. What kept me in the industry was the ability to be part of residents' lives, to bring moments of joy, to ensure they felt valued, respected, and still connected to life.

Looking back, I often think about the many times I was told I wouldn't succeed, from a Year 11 maths teacher to the clinical facilitators during my student days. Those voices could have shaped my path differently, but instead they became part of what drove me. I am proud of the way I have conducted myself, of the professionalism and integrity I have maintained, and of the values I have refused to compromise.

So, at the end of 2020, I applied for a Chief Executive Officer position at a small rural aged care organisation Edgarley Assisted Living. The Board took a chance on me and offered me the role.

Accepting that position came with significant personal sacrifice. It meant leaving my family home in Kilmore while my youngest son completed his secondary schooling, and moving away from my parents, who had also relocated there to support us and were beginning to experience declining health. It was not an easy decision, but it was an opportunity to lead an organisation into the future at a time when the industry itself was facing unprecedented change. The Royal Commission had just handed down its report, with 173 recommendations that would reshape aged care in Australia.

I commenced on the 12th of December 2020, and it did not take long to realise the scale of the challenge ahead.

In my first six months, I found myself navigating a deeply divided Board of Directors, with two clear factions and competing agendas. At the same time, I was stepping into a community where being "local" meant generations of connection. As someone new to the area, I was met with resistance, not only from some staff, but also from members of the community. There were moments of open scepticism, and at times, less subtle forms of exclusion. Social events were not always welcoming, and criticism often came from unexpected places.

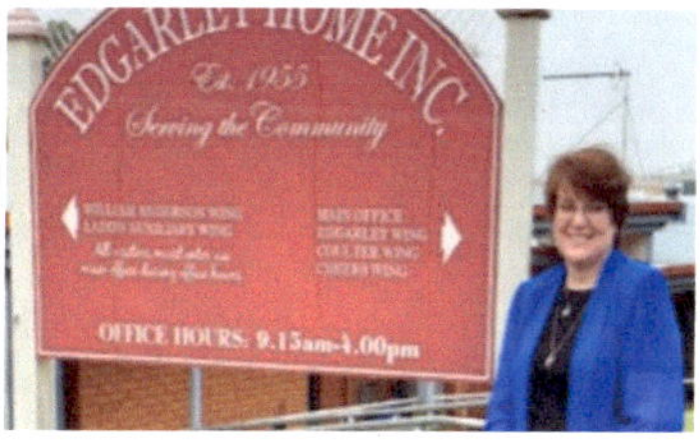

Despite this, I made a conscious decision to step outside my comfort zone and engage.

Within my first year, I submitted a project through a local council fundraising initiative, a Shark Tank pitch to a virtual crowdfunding event. Our vision was to build a playground on site to encourage intergenerational connection. It was about more than equipment; it was about bringing life, laughter, and community into the home. The project was successful, raising over $10,000, and marked an important step in building both trust and momentum.

At the same time, the organisation had already commenced a significant redevelopment project. The existing 43-bed facility was being transformed into a 60-bed home, a process that would take until September 2023 to complete. Managing this alongside day-to-day operations required careful planning, resilience, and a willingness to adapt constantly as challenges arose.

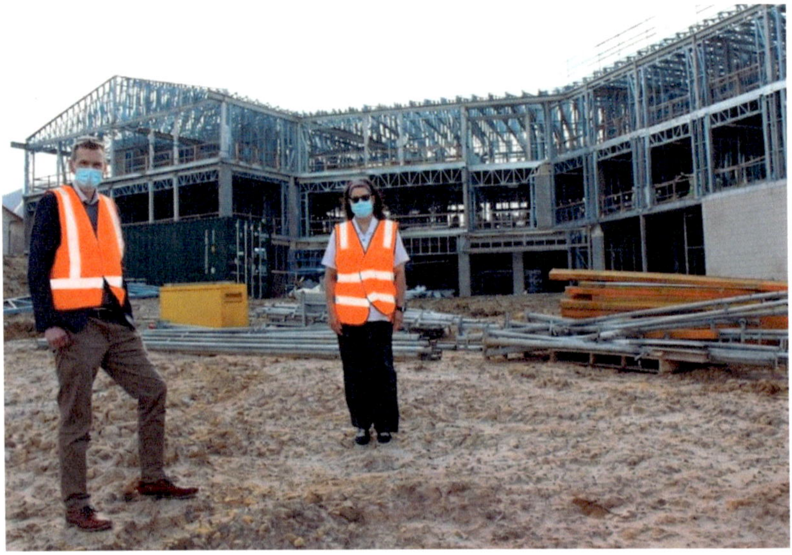

In 2021, I committed to further developing my leadership skills by enrolling in a CEO certification course online through the University of New England. It took longer than anticipated to complete, impacted by both work commitments and a major personal crisis, but by the end of 2024, I had achieved certification. It was not just an academic milestone, but a personal one, a reminder that growth does not stop, regardless of where you are in your career.

Throughout this time, staffing challenges remained a constant. Like many rural facilities, we experienced shortages of registered nurses, and it was not uncommon for me to step back onto the floor, working two to four RN shifts within a fortnight. For me, this was never about filling gaps, it was about showing the team that leadership is not confined to an office. It is about standing alongside your staff, understanding their challenges, and sharing the workload when needed.

The culture within the home continued to evolve, shaped by both intentional initiatives and the personalities that filled it. We embraced the presence of animals, recognising the comfort and connection they bring. Over time, we have had fish, birds, and four cats. One cat arrived uninvited, wandering in from a neighbouring property and deciding to stay. Another came with a resident who would not enter care without it. These small additions brought warmth and familiarity into the environment, reinforcing that this was not just a facility, but a home.

Staff morale was equally important. Dress-up days became a regular occurrence, bringing humour and energy into the workplace, along the Eden Philosophy guidelines. On one occasion, even the local doctor joined in, arriving in a full tiger costume. These moments, while simple, helped strengthen relationships and reminded everyone that care environments do not have to be devoid of joy.

In October 2024, the town was hit by a severe storm, blanketing the area in hail and causing widespread damage estimated at $55 million. Our newly built facility was not spared, requiring a complete roof replacement. Inside the facility rooms flooded with some holding more than an inch of water. Residents had to be relocated quickly, often under stressful conditions. One resident, when asked to leave her room, simply looked at us and said, "Just give me a broom, I can fix it." It was a moment that captured both the resilience and the character of the people we cared for.

The residents themselves continued to shape my experience. One gentleman, a local identity and former motorcycle racer from the 1940s, would share stories of his younger years racing bikes with sidecars, navigating bends by putting a foot to the ground. Whether entirely accurate or slightly embellished, his stories were part of the fabric of the home. Alongside his two lifelong friends, also residents, the "boys" brought humour, mischief, and a sense of continuity to the environment, often flirting harmlessly with staff and keeping everyone entertained.

Operationally, the organisation underwent significant transformation. When I commenced, systems were largely paper-based, and staffing numbers sat between 43 and 50 employees. Today, we employ close to 100 staff across a range of roles, including registered and enrolled nurses, personal care workers, catering, domestic, maintenance, and even our own physiotherapist. Technology has been introduced to streamline processes, improve documentation, and enhance overall efficiency.

I have also sought to strengthen the organisation's connection to its history and community. We engaged a young local author to document the story of the home, which was originally established in 1956 following the donation of a house to the community. Over the decades, it has experienced significant events, from security lockdowns to union disputes and major redevelopment, but its core purpose has remained unchanged: to serve the community.

Community engagement has remained a priority. We have participated in fundraising initiatives, including challenges to support the Royal Children's Hospital, where residents contribute and, in return, I subject myself to various activities, cream pies, ice baths, and whatever else the team decides. At Christmas, we introduced an annual "reindeer hunt," where staff, wearing antlers, move between designated spots while residents armed with water guns attempt to "take them down." What often begins as a simple activity frequently escalates into full-scale water fights, blurring the lines between staff and residents in the best possible way.

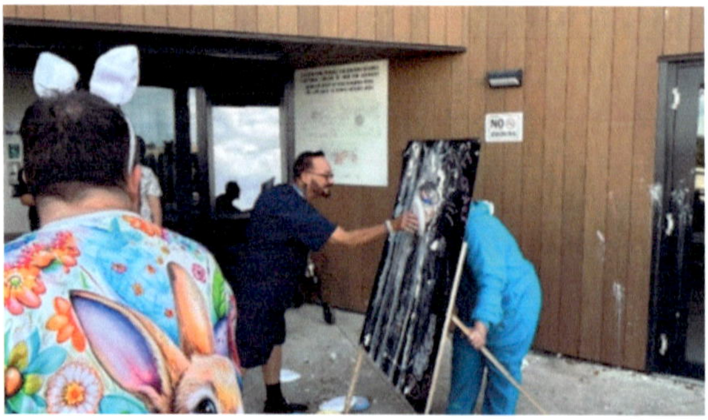

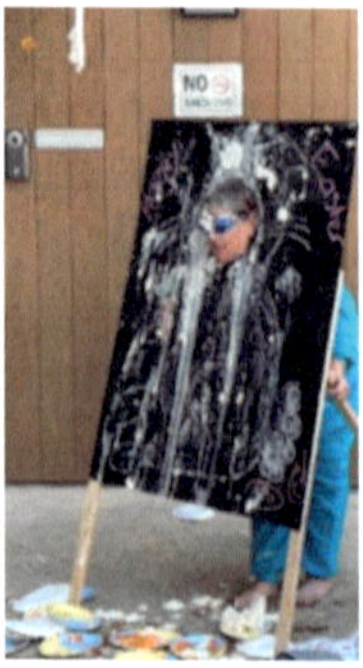

One of the more significant challenges faced by the community was the loss of its only local doctor, leaving the town without consistent medical coverage for nearly eighteen months. Through discussions with a visiting locum, an opportunity emerged and I convinced him that by using vacant space within our facility, he could establish his own practice, restoring access to local healthcare. It was a reminder that sometimes solutions come not from systems, but from conversations and relationships.

As regulatory changes introduced minimum staffing requirements, the organisation had to explore international recruitment to remain compliant. This brought with it a new layer of complexity, including visa processes, union negotiations, and labour agreements, areas I had never anticipated becoming so familiar with.

In recent years, my focus has also shifted towards giving back to the industry. Edgarley partnered with regional education provider Southwest TAFE to support the development of a Clinical Skills Bus, designed to enhance training opportunities for Certificate III personal care students in regional areas. The initiative was recognised by the state government with a Victorian Education and Skills Award, highlighting the impact that collaboration and innovation can have on workforce development.

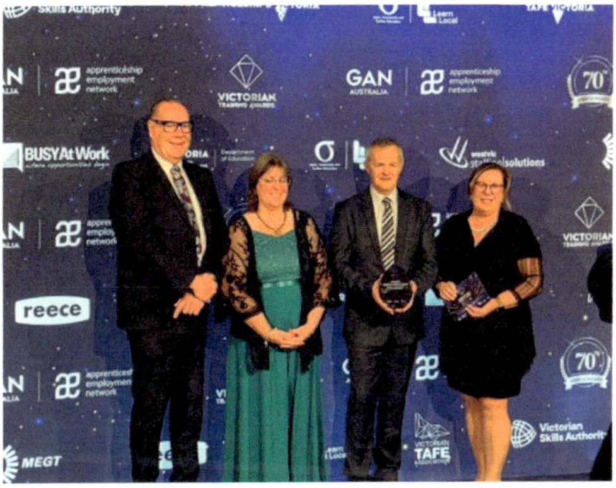

The winner of the Industry Collaboration Award at the 2024 Victorian Training Awards
SWTAFE – Mobile Skills Lab - Aged Care Collaboration.
This initiative, developed by South West TAFE alongside industry partners Eventide, Edgarley Assisted Living, Calvary Community Care, and Mulleraterong, provides a simulated, mobile aged care workplace to train remote learners.

I have also continued to engage with the broader industry, presenting at conferences, facilitating panel discussions, and sharing insights from my experiences. These opportunities have allowed me to contribute in a different way, not just through practice, but through influence and knowledge sharing.

While no organisation or individual is perfect, I can say with confidence that the level of care within Edgarley is one I would trust for my own parents. That, for me, is the benchmark that matters most.
The challenges facing small rural providers, however, continue to grow. Increasing staffing requirements, rising costs, and expanded regulatory expectations place significant pressure on organisations. Boards seek answers around financial sustainability, while at the same time, expectations around quality, infrastructure, and services continue to increase. From upgraded furnishings to additional software systems, from staffing ratios to documentation demands, the cost of care continues to rise.

Yet despite these pressures, the purpose remains unchanged.

Edgarley was established in 1956 to serve its community, and that mission continues to guide everything we do. It has evolved, adapted, and grown over the decades, but its foundation remains the same. As long as I remain in this role, I will continue to advocate for its future, to ensure it not only survives, but thrives, for the generations to come.

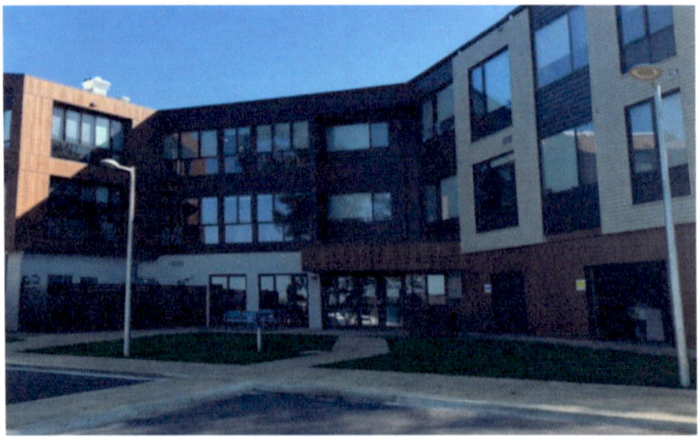

Why It Still Matters and Where We Stand Now

There are still many who work in aged care not because it is easy, convenient, or financially rewarding, but because they genuinely care. They see nursing—particularly aged care—not as a job, but as a calling, and they arrive each day with a quiet understanding that what they do matters, even when it goes unseen or unrecognised. That truth has remained constant, even as almost everything else around it has changed.

When I first entered the industry, I had no vision of leadership and certainly no expectation that I would one day become a Chief Executive Officer. My thinking was simple and practical: I would work, step away to raise a family, and perhaps return later in some capacity. Leadership was not something I sought, nor something I believed I was suited for at the time. I still remember returning to work after having children and taking on my first agency shift, which also happened to be the day I was punched in the face. When I got home, my mother asked me how my day had been, and after I told her what had happened, she asked a simple question: "Do you want to go back?" My answer was yes—not because the day had been easy, but because it had been meaningful. For the first time in years, I had been part of something beyond my immediate world, I had spoken with adults, I had been listened to, and I had felt that what I contributed mattered.

Even then, I did not see myself as a future leader. The negative voices from earlier years, the teacher who said I would not amount to anything, the clinical facilitators who doubted my ability, had not disappeared entirely. They lingered in the background and surfaced at times, causing me to question whether I truly had what it took, not only to be a good nurse, but to progress any further. What I did come to understand quite clearly, however, was the type of leader I did not want to become. I had witnessed leadership that relied on criticism rather than guidance, control rather than trust, and authority rather than respect, and I saw the impact this had on staff morale, retention, and ultimately on the quality of care delivered. These experiences shaped my thinking just as strongly as the positive ones that would come later.

Fortunately, I also encountered leaders who demonstrated a very different approach, individuals who showed that effective leadership is grounded in empathy, consistency, and the ability to bring out the best in others. They understood that leadership is not about position, but about influence, and not about hierarchy, but about trust. What they taught me, both directly and by example, was that to lead well you must genuinely care, not only about outcomes and organisational performance, but about the people who deliver that care every single day. This understanding became the foundation of my own leadership approach, shaping how I engaged with staff, how I made decisions, and how I held myself accountable to the same standards I expected of others.

As my role evolved from frontline care into management and eventually executive leadership, I gained something I had not previously had—the ability to influence change on a broader scale. This brought with it a sense of responsibility, but also opportunity. Early in that journey, I made a commitment to myself that if I was ever in a position to lead, I would never place finances ahead of people, and that the care provided would always reflect the standard I would expect for my own family. That principle has remained central to every decision I have made, even as the environment around me has become increasingly complex.

Over the past thirty years, aged care has undergone continuous reform, and while much of this change has been driven by a genuine desire to improve outcomes, it has also introduced layers of complexity that have reshaped the way care is delivered. Funding models have transitioned from RCI to ACFI and now to AN-ACC, each bringing new classifications, new processes, and, at times, a growing sense that clinical judgement is being replaced by systems of validation and external oversight. Alongside these changes has been the introduction of increasingly complex financial arrangements, RADs, DAPs, and DACs—which have made it more difficult for residents and families to clearly understand what they are paying for and why.

For more than a decade, aged care has been described as being "in crisis," and while the Royal Commission brought necessary attention to long-standing issues within the sector, it also accelerated a shift toward increased regulation, reporting, and compliance. Many of these reforms were well-intentioned and aimed at improving safety and accountability; however, the practical impact has been significant, particularly for providers operating with limited resources. The introduction of minimum staffing requirements with expanded documentation obligations and heightened compliance expectations has placed considerable pressure on organisations already navigating workforce shortages and financial constraints.

Funding has not kept pace with these increasing demands, and the cost of meeting regulatory expectations continues to rise. Employing additional registered nurses, achieving mandated care minutes, upgrading facilities, implementing new systems, and maintaining compliance all require substantial investment, and for many providers, particularly those in regional and rural areas, this pressure is ongoing and, at times, unsustainable. At the same time, the administrative burden placed on staff has grown to the point where documentation and reporting can begin to overshadow the delivery of care itself, raising an important and often uncomfortable question about where the balance truly lies.

At the centre of all of this are the residents, who are not concerned with funding models, regulatory frameworks, or compliance metrics, but with dignity, comfort, and human connection. Yet we now find ourselves in a system where elements that were once considered fundamental, such as personal comfort and quality of life, can be classified as additional services. This shift raises broader questions about how we define care and whether, in some areas, the system has moved too far away from its original purpose.

Despite these challenges, the majority of aged care providers and staff continue to deliver care with dedication and integrity. However, public perception has been shaped by the actions of a minority, and the sector as a whole has often been judged through that lens. At the same time, significant investment has been directed toward auditing, monitoring, and policy development, frequently at a distance from the realities of frontline care. While oversight is necessary, it does not replace the insight that comes from lived experience, nor does it automatically translate into improved conditions for those delivering care on a daily basis.

Workforce shortages remain one of the most pressing issues facing the sector, with experienced staff leaving due to burnout, increased pressure, and the lasting effects of the COVID-19 pandemic. Replacing them is not straightforward, as aged care has long struggled with its perception as a less desirable area of practice, and current conditions are making recruitment and retention even more difficult. The need for skilled, compassionate staff is immediate, yet the pipeline to develop and sustain that workforce is not keeping pace.

There is also an emerging gap in leadership, as experienced clinicians and managers retire and fewer individuals are prepared to step into these roles. Leadership in aged care requires a combination of clinical knowledge, resilience, adaptability, and strong interpersonal capability, and these qualities are not always prioritised in traditional training pathways. As a result, the sector risks losing not only its workforce, but also the experience and guidance that underpin effective leadership.

Looking ahead, the challenges facing aged care cannot be addressed through a single solution or policy change. They require a coordinated and practical approach that includes education and training, sustainable funding, workforce support, and a deliberate shift in how the profession is valued and understood. Equally important is the recognition that so-called "soft skills", empathy, communication, and the ability to connect are not secondary to clinical ability, but central to the delivery of meaningful care, and must be actively developed and supported.

Aged care, at its core, remains a deeply human profession, offering a level of connection and purpose that is difficult to replicate elsewhere. There is still an opportunity to rebuild, to restore balance, and to create a system that better supports both those receiving care and those providing it. However, time is not on our side. An ageing population will place increasing demand on a system already under pressure, and without timely, practical action, the gap between need and capacity will continue to grow.

The path forward requires more than continued review or additional layers of regulation. It requires decisions informed by the lived experience of those working within the sector, a willingness to reduce unnecessary complexity, and a commitment to refocus on what matters most. Because beyond every framework, every reform, and every discussion, there is a person at the centre of it all, and they deserve more than a system struggling to keep up.

This has always been, and will always remain, about people. And that is why, despite everything, this work still matters,

because care matters.

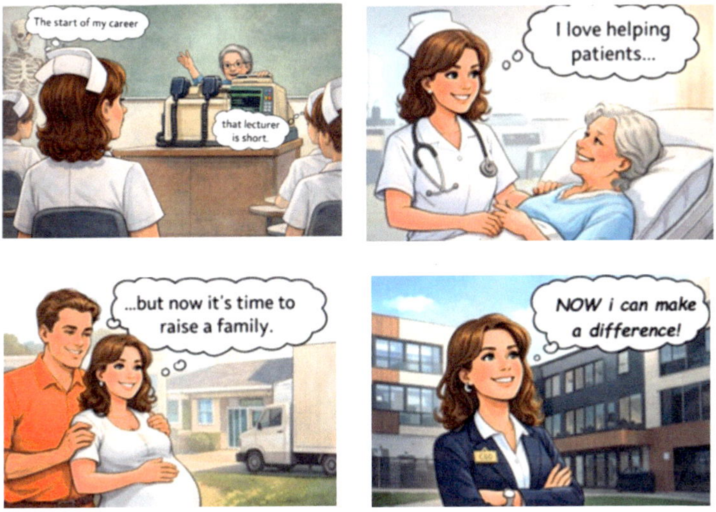

About the Author

Susan Wray is a Registered Nurse with over 35 years of experience, including nearly 27 years dedicated to aged care. For the past 14 years, she has held leadership roles in management, guiding teams through the complex and often challenging realities of delivering care in an evolving healthcare system.

She is deeply passionate about quality care for older Australians, with a strong focus on palliative care and preserving dignity at the end of life. Susan is also a committed advocate for the ongoing education and development of staff, believing that well-supported caregivers are essential to achieving meaningful, compassionate care.

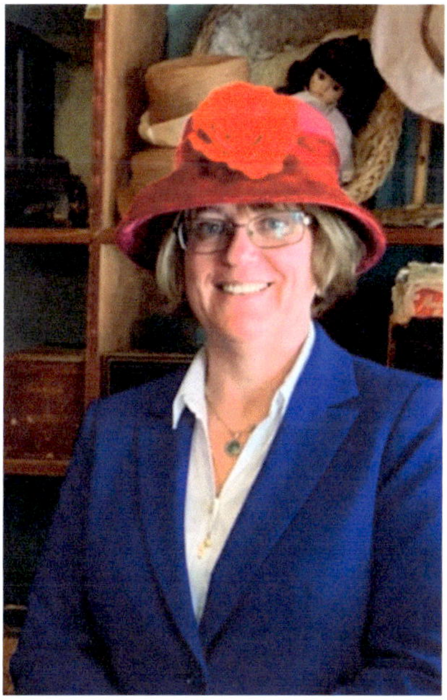

Beyond her clinical career, Susan has been a volunteer AFL football medic for over 30 years, supporting players from junior levels through to the VFL. She has also presented at numerous national conferences on aged care, sharing her experience, insights, and commitment to improving the sector.

Susan is married with three children. Drawing on a lifetime of both professional and personal experience, she brings authenticity, insight, and compassion to her writing, offering readers a rare and honest perspective on what it truly means to care.